About the author

Gareth is quite a large man with self-confessed, addictive behaviour. Thankfully after some near-death encounters, he managed to focus that into learning. When he's not training or treating clients, Gareth can be found drinking coffee while glued to his laptop, eating or having a friendly game of who can strangle who at his local Brazilian jujitsu school. In his time, he has trained people from all walks of life, including helping a world champion kick boxer to win two world titles as well as preparing many Mixed Martial Arts fighters for the cage. He has treated a ton of people for pain, movement problems, vertigo, insomnia, anxiety, pelvic floor issues and more. Although Gareth can be a bit of a potty mouth, he does it with love in his heart.

Foreword

.

To say that Gareth Riddy is a creative genius in his work as: a neurologic practitioner, a movement specialist, a trainer, a therapist & just in his daily pursuits as an all round good guy is both true & clearly obvious to anyone who's been involved with him in these fields.

It is impossible however to be consistently both creative and successful if one lacks the knowledge & understanding of their chosen field, to be able to apply their genius creatively. Gareth truly is that creative genius, but look beyond: his witty insights, his amusing anecdotes, even his manipulation of the vernacular and you will find a deeper knowledge and understanding of not just human physiology, but also the interplay between the hardwiring of human neurophysiology and all of the deeper intangibles within us that piece together what it is to be an intelligent, emotional, functional & healthy human being, negotiating our way through a mine field of the potential stresses that the modern day human being is faced with.

Gareth's mission is to empower people with the knowledge & the tools necessary to alleviate themselves of the harmful effects of modern day life on both their short and their long-term health. In the health and wellness industry, there are many who speak & few who are worth listening to. Gareth is one of those few.

Enjoy!

Scott Robinson – Applied Movement Neurology, Master practitioner & long time admirer of Gareth's impressive work with those who come to see him.

How to undo the shit the modern world does to us

Gareth Riddy

Intro

Hello Kiddywinks,

Welcome to my book. Thanks for giving me a go. I hope you find something of value. This is a collection of things that I have learned in my quest to help people, including myself, live a healthy, happy life in this rather fucked up modern world.

With well over a decade of experience working in the health and fitness industry, seventeen years as nightclub doorman and a spot of homelessness and drug addiction before that, I have learned some quite useful lessons. In the spirit of caring and sharing, I am here to give those lessons to you. Each one is important if you want to move forward, be healthy, happy and live a life of purpose, rather than being swept up and dragged down by the bullshit.

As the modern world moves on, it has certain expectations of us, or so we think. Those expectations take us further away from these things, these truths. It takes us further away from what it is to be human. That only ends in unhappiness, poor health, feeling trapped in your body and your mind and not getting the most out of your life.

The modern world is hazardous but there is no getting away from it. We all need to learn how to deal with the world we live in, if we want to thrive. As a human being we have certain innate physiological and psychological needs. They must be honoured despite what the modern world expects. Do that and you shall thrive.

I have managed to squeeze each point rather clumsily into the letters of my name, purely because it made me laugh. In the spirit of basically entertaining myself, I decided to call the system 'Life is Better with Gareth'. That is only funny if you know me though, so I decided to call the book something completely different instead.

It is my mission to undo the shit the modern world does to us. Everything I do has that one thing in mind.

Big punkass love

Chapter 1: My Life

In the beginning...

Let me tell you a little bit about myself so you have an idea where I'm coming from and if I may have anything of value to say. When it comes to health and happiness, with well over a decade working in the health and fitness industry, there should be at least something—I hope so anyway.

I was born five weeks premature at just over four pounds. There were some complications, so I needed to be incubated for a few days and fed through a tube up my nose until they got me up to a safer weight. Not the greatest of starts, but not the worst either. My mum and dad split very early on and we became a single parent family, back before it was fashionable. We were pioneers.

When I was about three or four we found out I was badly asthmatic, again before it was fashionable. Pioneering again. The asthma plagued me for years, and I have been in and out of hospital all through my life. It is still there but controlled, thankfully, as I have a better understanding of myself and my health. Unfortunately, the asthma meant I wasn't very active as I couldn't do all the stuff normal kids do, at least not as well. When I did try it always ended up with me collapsing into a wheezy mess and needing my inhaler.

Unsurprisingly, being inactive did lead to me being a bit on the porky side and I developed an unhealthy relationship with food early on. Something I partly learned from my mum but also something I did because I was so unhappy. I wasn't like the other kids—I was frail, fat and I felt isolated. From a very early age I had developed some self-limiting beliefs.

Fast-forward to my early teens and those limiting beliefs had grown along with me. I still wasn't like the other kids. I was painfully shy and to make matters worse I was very tall for my age, as well as overweight, so I attracted attention. The worst thing for a shy person. My unhealthy relationship with food was basically a search for somewhere to hide.

That search eventually led me to drugs. They became my best friend, they made feel different and I could be different. They enabled me to build this kind of crazy persona which masked how I really felt. Long story short, I did a lot of drugs, of all kinds. You name it, I did it, always to excess. My love affair with drugs eventually led me to homelessness and doing the whole squatter and traveller site thing for a while. When I was eighteen years old and living on one of the sites, a farmer came to visit. He was wielding a shotgun rather insistently and, in a strangely persuasive manner, asking us to leave his land.

My scared inner child reared his head and I shit myself, not literally, thankfully. That was me well and truly persuaded. I walked a couple of miles to the nearest phone box and phoned my grandparents, who thankfully took me in. If it wasn't for them I am convinced I would not be alive to tell the tale. Living with them meant I wasn't around all the heroin and I had a sanctuary. Slowly but surely, I began to move away from that life. Within a year I was completely out of it and drug free… OK, that's a bit of a lie—I smoked weed consistently until my late twenties. Still, it was very different ball game to all the class A's and it wasn't life consuming, as much.

Learning on my feet

The first job that I ever managed to hold down for more than a couple of weeks, mainly because it didn't involve me getting up early, was a nightclub doorman. Considering the level of fear and shyness I felt all throughout my life, it was a pretty strange career choice. Somehow it worked though. It was sink or swim and I didn't drown, although I felt like I was drowning a lot of the time. One of the wonderful things about that job is that it stopped me from getting out of my face, as it's a damn good idea to have your shit together if you have to deal with violence on a regular basis. So, I could only do things like that after work or on my days off. It helped me immensely. For seventeen years on and off I was in that game. It taught me a lot about myself, that I could hold my nerve when things got crazy, when all I really wanted to do was run away. That was a feeling I never got used to.

The funny thing is it wasn't those crazy situations that were the worst. When they happened, you didn't really have time to think. I remember a particularly large dance floor brawl with a pile of bodies scrapping on the floor, surrounded by more people kicking and stamping on them. The scene was chaotic and growing by the second. When something like that happens, you are running on instinct. From my vantage point, I saw the dance floor suddenly erupt in violence. I made the call on the radio and ran straight in, hoping I wouldn't be on my own when I got there. Thankfully I was joined by another doorman, Fred. He was a veteran like me, we had worked together many times over the years. I knew he had my back and he knew I had his. As we were so outnumbered, we couldn't just try to restrain a couple of them or we would have been swarmed. All that kicking and stamping would have been aimed at us.

We set to work, going from the outside in. Dragging people off and throwing them aside. When we got to the middle we realised we had surrounded ourselves. In a scene that must've looked like something out of a film, we immediately went back to back and got our hands up ready to start throwing. The crowd around us were shouting and swearing and trying to gear themselves up to attack but nobody wanted to be the first in. They knew we were ready. In the psychology of a mob, it just takes one and they all jump in. Thankfully during that momentary lull, the rest of door team appeared and people started getting dragged out. We were so lucky—had someone had the balls to be the first in and set the rest off, there is no way Fred or me would've come out unscathed.

After that I got asked several times by different people who saw the whole thing if I was scared. The answer was "No, I didn't have time, I was a bit busy". The whole incident probably took less than two minutes. The most stressful incidents were those that you knew, or thought, were coming. Anticipation is a killer, particularly if nothing does happen, leaving you with all those stress hormones floating around with nowhere to go. This is true in all walks of life. It is this thinking about things that may never, and often don't, happen that is damaging. Particularly when people don't do things to get rid of those stress hormones. This is one of the reasons exercise is so important. The two most important things that I learned from that job were patience (something which, luckily, I have in abundance) and getting comfortable with being uncomfortable. Two very valuable life skills.

Hitting the gym

Early on in my door career, I had a problem. It was one that I tried ignoring but it nearly got me, and those around me, in trouble more than once. I had to take notice. The problem was my asthma. After physically throwing somebody out, I would often need my inhaler. If the altercation went on, I sometimes needed to step back or hide in the office to take my inhaler and then get straight back out to it. Obviously, that was less than ideal, and I didn't always have the option to just step out if things were really kicking off.

At that time, the place I worked was the roughest in town. A place where taxi drivers refused to pick people up. We were on an industrial estate sandwiched between two of the rougher areas of town. We had all the naughty shitbags from the local estates, that had been barred from the town centre pubs and clubs. Not only that, we were isolated. When there are other venues about, the doormen all look out for each other, so if one venue gets out of hand, the others arrive to help. It's an unwritten rule of door work. We didn't have the luxury of it here. To add to our isolation further, we had no police about like they did in town. There was no chance of them ever arriving before an incident was over. You get the idea, it was rough and not the place for me to be taking inhaler breaks. So I decided to join a gym and get fitter.

From the start, I loved the gym and I couldn't believe I had never done it before. The weight dropped off. I went from nineteen down to seventeen stone, got much stronger and rarely needed my inhaler mid-fight. Pretty quickly I decided I wanted to become a personal trainer. It was an exciting time, the dawn of the new millennium. I was twenty-four and had been training for about a year at this point. One of the trainers at the gym had suggested some courses and I quickly found one I wanted to do. My gran said she would help me with the cost, which was lovely of her. That woman has helped me more than she realises over the years.

Health woes

My body had a different idea of what I would be doing that year. I had a strange cyst come up on my throat. It looked like I had mumps but only on one side. Imagine somebody had cut a tennis ball in half and stuck it just under my jawline on one side. When I went to get it checked out, the doc lanced it and sucked out all sorts of goo. He said he would book me in for roughly six weeks' time to get the last stubborn bit taken out under general anaesthetic.

This was the first time I'd ever had surgery and I was more than a little nervous. My first experience of general anaesthetic was pretty cool though, I'm a big fan. When I woke up I found that I had a three-inch scar on my throat. "That's a big scar for small bit of cyst, how cool is that?" I thought to myself. I also had a tube stuck in there that was draining stuff out into a container that I had to carry about. Once I realised I was OK to move about, I chucked some clothes on, went for a piss and to make a joint in the toilet and then went outside to sit on the grass and smoke some weed. Getting stoned with anaesthetic wearing off was a first for me, I had a lovely time. "Operations are great," I thought to myself. When I got back to the ward I had quite a pissed off doctor and nurse waiting for me. They told me off like a naughty child for not telling them I was going somewhere, whoops. During the whole healing process, I kept playing with my scar, pulling it about. I didn't want it to heal cleanly, I wanted a big scar and I got my wish, sweet. Mature of me, I know. When it came time to take the stitches out, I didn't bother going to the hospital, I did it myself. Any excuse to be a bit naughty. It's safe to say that I have a rebellious streak. I wasn't completely naughty though, I did make the effort to go to my follow up appointment.

When I got there, I sat down at the doctor's desk and he said, "Surprise, you've got cancer." Maybe he didn't say that exactly, the words were a blur. My world suddenly folded inwards, my peripheral vision disappeared and I felt like I was inside a bubble. All the colour drained away from my vision. I couldn't see, I couldn't hear, I couldn't think. My head was spinning, I felt sick and numb. What a head fuck. Nobody had come with me as it was just a routine thing, or so we thought. So I got the bus home on my own. That felt like the longest bus journey of my life. It was actually only about fifteen minutes.

My head was full of questions. Am I going to die? Will I go bald? How do I tell my girlfriend, my friends and family? Telling my family was by far the worst thing. Again, I don't really remember the words. Just the faces, the emotions and the tears. Once that was done and settled (OK maybe not settled), I had to have another operation to find and remove the source. They had found that the cancer started in one of my tonsils and spread inwards. If it wasn't for that cyst coming up, I would never have known until it was too late. Thanks cyst.

This operation wasn't as fun, but I still went outside and got stoned afterwards—I thought 'fuck it' at this point. After the operation I went through six weeks of radiotherapy which is basically being slowly burned. It's like having a long X-ray, and completely painless during the treatment. The pain accumulates over time afterwards. I don't think I felt much for the first week, that soon changed. By the end of treatment, I had lost three stone in weight. Eating had become so painful due to the accumulating burns inside my mouth and throat. Now that was a life changing experience if ever I had one. Years later, I found out from my mum (as she became friends with the doctor) that I was the youngest person ever to have that type of cancer and I'm used as a case study in textbooks to this day. Told you I was a pioneer.

My treatment and recovery threw a spanner in the works, as it took quite some time to get back into training again. Over the course of maybe a couple of years I had got into some bad habits—still not exercising and eating crap. I think I was just pleased I could eat food again. It was catching up with me. I had an asthma attack brewing, my breathing was getting steadily worse. Who'd have thought that lifestyle and health were linked? Go figure. Somebody should tell people that. In very typical fashion, I insisted on still trying to get stoned even though I couldn't breathe very well. That night I woke up in the middle of an attack. All I remember is telling my girlfriend at the time to call an ambulance as I grabbed my inhaler and got myself to the floor, as if that somehow would help. The next thing I knew I had the paramedics standing over me. All I remember saying to them is "I'm not going anywhere without my pants." (That's underpants to those of you that aren't from sunny England.) According to my ex-girlfriend, I wasn't breathing for five minutes and I was unconscious for forty-five minutes. There was a bit of knock on effect from the oxygen deprivation: for a couple of years after that I had some memory issues, which I found pretty frustrating, but thankfully they passed.

A new start

After getting back into the gym for a while I decided (once again) to study to become a personal trainer when I was twenty-seven. That journey led me to here, with well over decade of constant learning, growing and soul searching being my new drug of choice. I got totally addicted to learning and self-discovery. Not only did I have my own life experiences as motivation to drive me forward—not wanting to go back there—but I was also, and am still, very motivated by my mum. She was unhappy and unhealthy her whole life. One of life's victims, as much of herself as she was to circumstance. Her life culminated a few years ago in her being diagnosed with non-Hodgkin's lymphoma, a form of cancer, that eventually ended her days at fifty-nine years of age. She said to me very early on, "If anything can wrong with treatment, it will—it always does with me."

I knew at that moment she would not survive—classic victim mentality that ultimately became a self-fulfilling prophecy. Towards the end, her tumours grew so much that they changed the shape of her head, it was almost like she was wearing a crash helmet of cancer under her skin. The last couple of days of her life she was in so much pain, she was kicking and screaming, as much as someone can in a weakened state, in between heavy doses of morphine. Go quietly in her sleep she did not. I am so thankful that those last days were at home with the whole family. On her last day, I was by her bedside, just me and the nurse in the room. Mum started to snore strangely, the nurse said that this was the end and went downstairs to get the rest of the family. Her last breath was right there, just us, me and my mum, just like my childhood. She was already gone when the family came into the room. That is a moment I will cherish forever. I was happy her suffering was over, relieved, honoured that her last breath was with me and I was heartbroken all in one intertwined emotion.

Seeing my mum suffer her whole life is what drives me. I saw a life wasted and very nearly wasted my own. If I could bring myself this far then I could help other people too. Suffering doesn't have to be the way life is. Far too many things are just accepted as the way things are and people die without having really lived. That is a true tragedy. Fuck that shit, I can't accept that.

All that stuff is what brought me here to be the bloke writing this book. My days are spent helping people get the most out of themselves whether it be face-to-face in a gym or therapy room or from the other side of a laptop screen. Moving better, feeling better, living better.

Chapter 2: G

Grounding

Right shall we get on with the system? OK then, we will. This section is going to be on the letter G. For this letter I have chosen grounding, also known as barefoot earthing. There will be some other stuff chucked in here as well, but it's all related. Now, I know it sounds like some massive hippy crap but bear with me, it will make more sense by the end of this. Basically, this whole section is about giving the human organism what it needs, biologically, from the environment we live in. Although we have come a long way as species with all our technological advances, we are all still biological organisms. We have basic needs as organisms that technology cannot yet meet. If you want to live healthy and happy and be functioning at a higher level, then these needs must be met.

The earth is a big electromagnetic ball, and every living thing also has this quality. OK, not the ball quality, no need to be pedantic! But all life is bioelectric in nature. For the first sixteen days after conception, our cells are guided by this bioelectricity. It is how our cells multiply before our nervous system has started to develop. We are electricity before we are anything else. There is a constant flow back and forth between the earth and those living things that contact it, which is everything. There is one exception and that is us, in the western world, living our insulated lives. When our shoes became rubber, around the 1960s I think, we got cut off. We live in houses, drive cars and are surrounded by non-natural electromagnetic fields which leaves us disconnected and feeling fried. The earth is a source of free electrons and we aren't getting any.

Why do electrons matter? Well, funny you should ask. We've all seen pictures of atoms, right? Those dots that spin around the outside are electrons. Atoms lose electrons all the time in a process known as oxidisation. Now when an atom loses an electron, it becomes unstable and robs an electron off a neighbouring atom so that it can stabilise itself. The thieving little bastard. This then becomes a chain reaction of thievery that causes degeneration and cellular damage until every atom has enough electrons to become stable. The damage caused is what is known as free radical damage. It is why we need antioxidants in our diets, as they provide electrons in nutrient form. The earth also supplies it directly through the conductive nature of all livings things, which I'm guessing is how the fruit gets it in the first place...

That's the science bit over. Now I'm not sure if being grounded helps us relax or if a lack of grounding prevents us from relaxing, but either way the outcome is the same. Have you ever noticed how much more relaxed you feel when at the beach, or laying in the garden on a nice day? It makes a significant difference. There is a ton of science out there from scientists doing studies on this stuff if you're into that sort of thing, just google away. I might stick a link or two in for you if you're lucky. On a personal note, when I first discovered earthing I started playing with a blood pressure monitor, while grounded and not grounded. Every time I was grounded my blood pressure dropped, as did my pulse rate, straight away. You can also measure your body's voltage with a multimeter and see the difference, so it's very measurable in cold hard numbers.

I also started sleeping better which was something I hadn't done properly in over twenty years. So even if all it does is help you relax, sleep better and lower your blood pressure for a bit then it's a bloody good thing to do, and that shit's free! Why wouldn't you try it? All you need to do is make contact with the earth without your insulating shoes. Get barefoot, walk on the grass. Go touch a tree or a bush with your hands, basically contact anything natural and alive. I recommend aiming for a minimum of fifteen mins a day, although ultimately the more you can do, the better. After all, there was a time when, as a species, we were earthed constantly.

Now I know weather isn't always on our side with this, depending on your location. I'm in sunny England so it often isn't anyway. Luckily you can buy earthing gear easily on the internet. Mats, bedding, wristbands and sandals. These can be plugged into the mains and use the earthing point to do just that, earth. Personally, I prefer to plug my mat in outside, directly into the ground with a long wire. I find I feel better than if it's in the mains. My mat is on my bed so I sleep earthed, and it makes a massive difference. If I had to choose just one time to do it, I would say earthing yourself before bed is the way to start. First thing in the morning and just before bed is better. As much as you can is best.

Our environment

This next topic is a bit different but I lump this in together as it's still about our relationship with the environment. Light is the star of this show. Our natural biological rhythms are tied into the light and dark cycles of the earth. Day and night, awake and asleep. When it's dark, our brain registers this through the eyes. The body slows down and gets ready to take care of lots of important processes while we sleep. At this time, our thyroid is doing its thing, taking care of our metabolism. Our liver is super busy, dealing with how our body metabolises sugars and fats, dealing with stress hormones, helping to take harmful toxins out of our systems, and it also has a role in regulating our sex hormones. For you men out there, waking up without a tent pole is an indicator your hormones are not at a great level and you are not getting enough quality sleep. So get some sleep and stay hard! The liver has a lot to do and if we aren't asleep when we should be, it can't do its job properly.

Light

Not only is the liver busy, but our brains have some detoxing to do of their own, which also relies on being asleep. In particular, it relies on a hormone called melatonin to help this process. Melatonin is very much linked to light, or more accurately lack of light. Too much light at the wrong time means no melatonin. With all that in mind, it's easy to see how poor sleep is detrimental to our health and well-being. Lack of sleep has been linked to cardiovascular disease, diabetes, obesity, psychological illnesses, behavioural problems, Alzheimer's, memory, reaction time, and much more. In a nutshell your body can't run itself and repair properly without sleep. That can manifest itself in a whole lot of shit ways.

Not all light is created equal. We developed as inhabitants of this planet, with in the full spectrum of sunlight. Our problems in the modern world are twofold. One: we are not exposed to much sunlight and when we are, we're normally covered in sunblock which is actually blocking out the good stuff, or we're binging on sun and getting burnt. Problem number two is all the artificial light we are exposed to. Now light is a very big subject and this by no means covers everything. Among other things we have a big overexposure to blue light, far exceeding the amount that can be found naturally, within full spectrum sunlight. Blue light concentrations at their highest and most harmful come from backlit screens, so think smart phones, tablets, and PCs. You've no doubt seen that blue glow on someone when they're looking at their phone in the dark. Blue light in excessive amounts and at the wrong time is a right fucker.

First off, it is known for being a factor in macular degeneration, or as I like to say, it fucks your vision up. It also is hugely disruptive to our circadian biology. Circadian is just a science word for body clock. I have a theory that a lot of problems are going to come to light (pun intended) from kids being over exposed to screens, from having their circadian biology disrupted before they are even developed. All that light pouring into our eyes is signalling to our brain that it is day time and our brain will act accordingly. All the hormones and chemicals that should be up and about in the day will be doing their thing. Among those is cortisol which is known as a stress hormone. Its job is to get us up and moving in the early part of the day as well as helping us in times of threat by mobilising fuel from the body and ramping us up for "fight or flight". Cortisol is very important, at the right time, in appropriate amounts. It is not however, the friend of bedtime. Have you ever gone to bed only to find your mind is chattering away with worries, tasks that need doing, replaying events and playing events that haven't even happened? That is a sign that your cortisol is out of whack, doing its thing at the wrong time of day. What is the friend of bedtime is a little neurotransmitter called serotonin. That little puppy helps you relax and ultimately get to sleep. It is great at night time, however if your cortisol is out of whack, your serotonin will also be out of whack. There is a seesaw effect, which often means it is higher in the morning, making it a struggle to get up and feel alive. Not the best way to start and end your days. There is other stuff going on with neurotransmitters and hormones but I don't want to overcomplicate things and turn this into a science book. I just want you to get the general idea.

Serotonin

Serotonin is known by some as the happy hormone. When people go to the doctor and get a prescription for antidepressants, those pills are generally aimed at regulating serotonin production and uptake. Personally, I think medicating is rarely the answer, if ever. Depression is a sign that we have become far too removed from what our bodies need biologically. It is a symptom, a sign that something needs to change (as is all pain for that matter). There are two very big problems with our approach to health in the western world, politics aside. I'll try not too carried away here, as this shit fucks me right off. One is we look to medicate symptoms as opposed to find and address the cause. A symptom-based approach doesn't get to the root of the problem and actually solve the issue. The medications themselves often come with their own problems too. It's a fucking great business model though, keeping customers coming back for life.

The second major problem is that we wait until we feel shit. We wait until something goes wrong and then we look to the doctors to fix us, with that very same, symptom-based approach. We are not taught how to look after our own health. We are taught to be passive with our health, essentially victims with no control, looking to be saved by the doctor.

How's that working out for you? It nearly killed me, quite a few times, and I watched it kill my mum. Although I tried for many years to get her to take ownership of her health, she remained passive, looking outside for help and for something to blame. No parent takes advice from their child after all and vice versa obviously. That rant was pretty mild for me, well done Gareth.

Now back to the whole light thing. In a nutshell, too much light at the wrong times messes with your body clock and consequently your health. Keep that in mind.

Takeaway tips

Because I'm nice and the whole point of this book is to be helpful, I'm going to give you some tips to deal with this problem. The obvious thing to do would be to limit screen time but, in this day and age, it is far from practical. Yes, the modern world fucks us up but we still have to live in it—living in a cave just isn't option for most people. The first thing I would recommend is to get a blue light filter on all your back lit devices. There are a ton of apps available for this. Make sure that it is set for twenty-four hours a day, not just night time. There are physical filters available that go on the screen if you'd prefer. You can also get blue light blocking glasses which help your cause even more. I'm wearing a pair as I type this. Do your best to get some full spectrum light from the sun, particularly in the morning. Again, I understand that this isn't always practical as people work different times and the weather doesn't always help us out. If you can, get out there morning and/or evening. Your body needs it, in the eyes and on the skin. We've all heard about Vitamin D from the sun and how it is important for health so I don't think I need to go into that. When you're at home in the evening, get yourself away from screens as early as possible. Personally, my phone goes off before 8pm, any later than that and I'm in trouble. 7pm is even better. Start dimming the light, and switch to lamps or even candles in the evening. The brain needs to know it is night time so it can start winding down the body in preparation for sleep. Try to avoid eating too late, preferably before seven or as close to as possible. All the extra work from breaking down a meal can keep us awake and disrupt everything that should be going on when we sleep.

Anything electrical needs to be off in the bedroom, even that little red light on the tv can be disruptive. Personally, I don't think the bedroom is the place for a TV. The bedroom is a place for the three S's: Sleeping, Sex and Somewhere to keep your clothes. That includes switching your phone off and not charging it in your room. If you are leaving it alone for a couple of hours before bed that is plenty of time to charge it anyway. What's more important, Facebook or your health? If your phone is your source of alarm, then simply put it on airplane mode. Lastly, make sure you get up and go to bed at the same time each day, even on weekends. Every time you have a lie-in you're basically giving yourself a bit of jetlag and disrupting your clock. Your health and quality of life are being affected by that extra hour or two in bed. Now I understand we all have lives to lead. There will be times when we can't stick to those rules, social engagements etc. Life happens. These are general guidelines, but the more you can stick to them, the better, so do your best, but don't beat yourself up when something comes up that needs doing and gets in the way, we need to enjoy ourselves too. Just try to be selective, going out every week won't do you any good in the long term.

Chapter 3: A

Attention

OK so the next letter in my name is A. We are going with Attention and Awareness. The concept is very simple and can be applied to anything you do. The more attention you put into a task, the better quality it will be, simple. One of the problems of modern living is our attention is pulled in multiple directions, constantly. At work, people often have so many tasks to do that they end up doing very little. Busy and productive are not the same things. To be truly productive you need to be able to pay attention and that requires the mental space to be able to do it. It is unfortunate that most employers don't see this, they go with the more is better approach. It's no wonder so many people are overworked, stressed out and underperforming all at the same time. Space is so important for good work, for life in general. If you look at a piece of writing and took all the spaces out it would become a mess, and the same is true for music. People are no different, we need those spaces to allow information to settle, to make sense of things. Not just on a cognitive level, our health demands it too.

There are so many things after our attention, that the really important things don't get the attention they deserve.

Our whole lives are pretty much like that in fact. We always have our phones within arm's reach where people can contact us through text, email, social media or good old-fashioned phone calls. When people aren't contacting us and distracting us, we reach for the phone and distract ourselves. We end up giving a good portion of our lives to that little screen! That's not the only screen in our lives, although it is probably the most influential. We have laptops, PCs, tablets and of course that life-sucking big screen, the TV. Using these things isn't always mutually exclusive either, a lot of people will sit watching TV while using their laptop or tablet and be on their phone all at the same time. It's no wonder it's been said that the average human attention span is less than eight seconds these days, literally less than a goldfish. I've checked my phone three times just writing these few lines. The less attention we pay, the less we are able to pay. Use it or lose it. Quality relies on attention. I suppose I'd better give you some examples.

Everyday attention examples

Paying attention in my conversations was something I struggled with for a long time and I got constantly called up on it by friends. I think it was an offshoot from my doorman days where in all my interactions I had to be constantly aware of my surroundings in case shit kicked off. Having one ear in the conversation and my eyes somewhere else. Thankfully my door days are long gone and I can talk to people without having to run off and deal with fights. In our day-to-day relationships it is all too easy to stop paying attention. To fall into the trap of thinking about what we want to say next or about something entirely different, instead of being present in the interaction. How we relate to others then suffers as a result. We're not creating any depth of connection, it's just people taking it in turns to talk about their stuff while not really listening to the other. This can lead to us feeling disconnected from the world, despite being surrounded by family, friends and colleagues. Connection is something we crave as humans, it is a big part of what makes us human. So pay attention, stop checking your phone and truly listen to those people in your life. Be present, not just in body. Your relationships will be better for it.

Cooking is another great example of something that needs attention. The best meals come from someone that is paying attention, being present. You could cook the exact same meal twice but they could be very different, both in quality and in cooking experience. The meal prepared while being distracted with our thoughts or life in general is easily messed up. Maybe the ingredients get out of balance, the food gets over or under cooked. Stuff gets spilled, food gets dropped on the floor. Sometimes things go seriously wrong, there is an accident, you could cut yourself, burn yourself, something catches fire or you might slip on some of that spillage. Here's an interesting little fact: the majority of fatal accidents in the home happen in the kitchen. If ever there is a place to pay attention, it is the kitchen. This isn't just a practical issue, it is also about quality and creativity. Being creative in any sense requires attention, and a lack of attention means a lack of quality. I'm going to take that one step further and say that love is the secret ingredient of a great creation, whatever it is. I remember reading an article a fair few years ago, from the strength coach Charles Poliquin, who I used to follow when I was into that sort of thing. In this article he said that "love is the most powerful creative force in the universe." That phrase stuck with me and it's something I use probably every week in some way. The idea is that if you put your heart and soul into a creation, it will be better than if you didn't. That love will motivate you to go further for your creation than if it was some other motivation. We all know when something has been made from love, it stands out.

Being "in love"

As I'm talking about love, let's go into that a little deeper. I'm differentiating romantic love, the idea of being in love, from the verb 'to love': the action of giving someone or something love, of doing something with love. Being in love, or more accurately infatuated, is a transient feeling. It is a chemical process in the body, an extremely potent and intense process at that. It lasts maybe a couple of years if you're lucky, also known as the honeymoon period. We are led to believe by films, novels and fairy tales that it can last forever. Unfortunately, that is just not true. It is a dangerous myth that leads to much unhappiness in the world. People blame themselves or their partners when the honeymoon period inevitably fades. "I love you but I'm not in love with you" is an all too common phrase. They jump from one relationship to the next, always chasing that oh-so-intoxicating but temporary feeling.

This phase exists for evolutionary reasons: to bond a couple intensely while they procreate. It then disappears and the focus shifts onto child rearing. Once the honeymoon period is over, that is when a true loving relationship can be built. A relationship where two people genuinely relate, support and encourage each other's growth. They grow together. If you believe the hype and fall into the trap of thinking being "in love" is meant to be permanent, then your chances of ever being in a truly happy relationship are slim to none. You'll be chasing an illusion while missing out on the proper stuff, a happy relationship. Don't underestimate how important a happy relationship is. It doesn't matter how successful you are, if your home life isn't right, then your shit is broken and it will affect everything else.

Now here is the big kicker about falling in love. Just because you fall in love with someone, it doesn't mean that person is right for you, that you are right for each other. You can definitely fall in love with the wrong person, more than once. I've totally been there and I was left with a relationship of conflict, wondering what went wrong. Often people fall into the trap of believing their partner is "The One", so they rush into marriage before the honeymoon period is over, only to be left with a relationship that doesn't work. They either end up divorced, feeling like a failure, or they live the rest of their lives in a loveless marriage. Kids are often born into that environment and grow up learning from their parents that this is the way life is meant to be and the whole cycle begins for the next generation.

On a slight side note, staying in a loveless relationship for the sake of the kids, doesn't work. Kids aren't stupid, they know when people aren't happy, you can't fake it. All people do is ruin their own lives and give the kids a jaded view of the world growing up, thinking shit relationships are normal. There are no winners in that situation.

Back to the whole "in love" thing. I'm not saying it is bad or you should avoid it by any means. It is an amazing and important part of life—it helped the human race get this far after all! It is also what brought my good lady wife, Nicola (told you I mentioned you in the book) and I together Just over ten years ago. What I'm saying is "in love" should be honoured for what it is: beautiful and temporary. Love is built off the back of that, it requires work, care and attention. Love isn't something that just happens, love is active. I got a little side tracked there. Let's not forget this section is about attention. On with the show...

Movement and learning

Our movement is at its best when we pay attention. Smoother and more controlled. We don't trip over or bump into things if we're paying attention, which is a bonus. When an athlete, dancer or martial artist is in the zone, present with complete attention, they are at their best. Performing at a higher level doesn't work if you're thinking about other things. That counts for anything you do. Later on, I go into movement a bit deeper so I'll leave that there for now.

Let's say you're one of these people that likes lifting weights, as I am quite partial to. You will feel the benefits much more if you focus on feeling the exercise as opposed to just moving the weight up and down for the allotted number of reps. Your brain will be connecting much more to your muscles, which will make your body way more responsive, and you can do it a lower weight, saving a bit of wear and tear on the body. Now I know all you blokes want to be lifting as heavy as possible (not including strength athletes, that's their whole thing), I've been there. In my younger days I used to chase those high numbers.

One time I thought that wearing a lifting belt would save me from any less than stellar form while doing heavy deadlifts. A popping sensation and a warm feeling creeping across my lower back informed that I was wrong. Having to spend the next four days sitting upright to sleep (wishful thinking that it was sleep) and crawling to get around the house made sure that I didn't forget how wrong I was. It took me about a week to be able to walk upright without looking like I had shit myself and another week to be able to put my shoes and socks on comfortably. That was last time I deadlifted badly and I didn't rely on a belt again.

As a man who has spent many years in the weight room and well over a decade training people in the gym, trust me when I say just chasing those high numbers doesn't have much longevity. The body adapts, becomes tight and is very prone to injury and pain. I don't care how massive or ripped you are, if you can't bend down to tie your shoes or reach something off a high shelf then it doesn't mean shit. It's just cosmetic and when that eventually fades, which it will, you will be left with a knackered body that can't move properly. You will end up fucked for a lot longer than you are in shape for.

From a neurological standpoint, the more attention we pay to something, the more the brain lights up. Throw in a learning aspect and it starts to rewire itself in new ways as it learns. This is something called neuroplasticity which is a fancy way of saying the brain's ability to change. It used to be thought in scientific circles that the brain couldn't change once we became adults. I remember being taught this as a kid. Thankfully that has since been found not to be true. The concept of neuroplasticity has had massive implications on the future of people with traumatic brain injuries and stroke patients. When a part of the brain has become injured or stopped functioning like it should, it has been shown that neighbouring healthy parts of the brain can start to rewire and learn how to do the job of the injured or dead area. Attention and effort is key to make the most of this innate ability. There was a documentary made a few years ago that beautifully demonstrated this in real life. It is called "Ping Pong" and is about an over-eighties ping pong world championship. One of the ladies competing had been put in a home after a stroke as she had lost the use of pretty much half her body and could no longer speak. She needed constant care. During her time there, she started to learn ping pong for something to do. The act of learning this new skill not only gave her a sense of enjoyment and was all-important movement and exercise for her but it also helped her brain rewire. Over time she regained her function. Her motor skills came back, including her speech, and she ended up competing in the world championships. I won't tell you how she did just in case you decide to watch it. Anyway, the point is, through the attention required to learn a new skill, she changed her life—neuroplasticity in action. With that knowledge of neuroplasticity in mind we can change ourselves, our behaviours, our habits into almost anything we want. I don't know about you but I fucking love that idea. It changed my whole approach to life. A healthy brain is one that can make new connections and adapt. That is ultimately how we learn and grow.

Awareness

Now onto awareness. Attention and awareness can be interchangeable, I'm just splitting it up like this because I'm coming at awareness from a slightly different angle than performing practical tasks and neurological wiring. What I am talking about is conscious awareness and not getting lost in thought, the illusion of thought. Taking the time to connect to yourself and disconnect from all that chattering away in your mind. There have been many books written on this subject, so I'm going to give you a very condensed version of how I see this.

Your mind runs its narrative constantly, telling stories that are for the most part not true. It can be a bit of a shit-stirring dickhead and it will stitch you right up if you listen to it! Don't take it personally, this isn't about you. You are not your thoughts. Thoughts come and go, they are transient. They hold no power until you pay attention to them, giving them energy. OK so let's do a bit of an experiment so you can see what I mean. All I want you to do is put this book down, just for two minutes. Sit back and try to watch your thoughts as they float by, listen to what they say but don't attach yourself to what they say. Just observe. Are you ready? OK, I'll see you in two minutes……

Hello, welcome back! How was that then, did you notice that thoughts just seem to happen? Personally, my mind comes up with some right nonsense. I can be walking along minding my own business and my mind will start criticizing people around me that I've never met and have no idea about. And yet my mind has made up a little story in an instant! It might be criticizing me, doubting me or making me worry about what other people may think. Predicting the future is very common— my mind will make up scenarios that I may encounter or even arguments I may have and how I would react if a certain situation happened, which it almost never does. The dickhead isn't even any good at predicting the future! If I'm not careful and I listen to that crap I may end up stressed about something that hasn't even happened. My mind also loves hanging out in the past, trying to make me stressed about things that can't be changed. What a shit-stirring dickhead.

As you can see, the mind just runs along doing its own thing. Just because you think something, it doesn't mean it is true. The problem for most people is they don't know that and get caught up in the shit stirring. Understanding that thoughts, when left to themselves, are often far from accurate is the first step. The second step is learning to use your mind for tasks: learning, problem solving, whatever you're trying to achieve; and to disassociate with the automatic ramblings of your mind when you're not using it. Those ramblings will happen anyway, but the point is that you don't attach to the story and believe the bullshit. Learn to use your mind consciously, with awareness. This is essentially the essence of zen or as it's now marketed in the modern world, mindfulness. Transcendental meditation is all about that, just being and letting your mind do its thing while you don't attach to it. Yoga came about as a moving meditation for people that struggle to just sit still as holding positions in yoga forces you to be very present, in the moment.

Meditation

Meditation deserves a bit more props than a passing mention. There are so many benefits to including some sort of meditation practice in your life. Don't think it's just for hippies. It benefits everyone. Many of the top performers in the world in various fields are big proponents of meditation and its benefits. Here's a list of just a few: Oprah, Ray Dalio, who founded one the world's biggest hedge funds; Tony Robbins, Hugh Jackman, Martin Scorsese, and Paul McCartney.

Those people, and many, many more, say that meditation helps keep them functioning at a higher level. It has been a big part of martial arts throughout history. The samurai were known for it. It enabled them to remain calm in the midst of battle, which is bloody good idea. Keeping calm in chaos was quite literally a matter of life and death for them. Being able to remain calm when things are going to shit is an awesome life skill, one we should all have. The chaos will come in life, so learn to embrace the chaos.

When you meditate, you are creating space for your mind and body. Space is crucial for growth. In weight training it is the resting where you repair and get stronger. If you didn't rest, you would just keep on breaking yourself down until eventually you got injured or ill. The principle is the same with the mind, we need space to repair and grow. On a cognitive level, meditation increases the ability to focus. Memory improves, as does problem solving and your creative thinking prowess. Emotionally, it lessens anxiety, stress and worry, increases optimism, your mood improves, resilience in general goes up and a biggie, it increases acceptance. One of the major sources of stress and unhappiness is people not being able to accept something that can't be changed. Acceptance is so important, without it you can't move forward in life. From a health perspective, meditation helps keep blood pressure down, lessens inflammatory issues and helps the immune system do what it should do. In short, meditation is cool as fuck.

Accepting responsibility

I've decided to stick another A in here. It's a very important topic that I originally left out and was going to save for another time. Some of my test audience for the original audio of this said it was a bit short so that was all the excuse I needed to put this in. You can thank them for it.

This A is for Accepting responsibility, for everything in your life, good and bad. Owning your shit. Culturally we are blamers, we are actively encouraged in fact. The problem with blame is it takes the responsibility from you and puts it onto something external, maybe even something that doesn't exist. When you blame, you are giving that thing responsibility over your problems, you are giving it power, your power. It is an act of passivity, being passive in the outcome of your life. Without responsibility, there can be no action, just reaction. Reacting is no way to live your life—that is just you being at the mercy of events. It's the difference between having a clear direction and being like a pinball.

People that do not take responsibility, do not own their shit, they blame. They blame outside forces for their problems. They blame parents, siblings, the education system, the neighbourhood, the government, Donald Trump's wig, Kim Jong Un's hair-cut, the banks, the Illuminati, pharmaceutical companies, aliens, the health service, the economy, religions, being born poor, being born rich... they can blame anything other than take responsibility themselves. Playing the blame game is ultimately disempowering. Every time you blame something, you are taking away your ability, your response ability, to change the situation. You are being a passive victim. It prevents you from learning from a situation and moving forward. Now I know bad things happen in life and sometimes they can't be avoided. Maybe it was something completely out of your control, you could have grown up with abuse or a drug-addicted parent, lost a limb in an accident or whatever. My point is if you spend your time blaming that situation, you are not spending your time moving beyond it. Life happens, it's how you deal with it that makes the difference.

Let me tell you a story of someone that let go of blame and did reasonably well for it. This is a lady who was born in the early fifties in America, she was born black, which in that era was setting you up for a proper shit time straight off the bat, as the civil rights movement was only just beginning. Not only that, being female came with its own issues. In those days a woman's place was in the home. Those that did have jobs mainly did things like school teaching, factory work or secretarial work. There were very few women in relative higher positions. Women just didn't have the same opportunities for careers as men, they pretty much didn't have careers full stop. It was a very different time. She grew up with sexual abuse and violence. At fourteen years old she had a baby from abuse and that baby did not survive past infancy. There were plenty of drugs in her life as she got older too. Now that lady today in 2017 is considered one of the most powerful women in America, is worth three billion dollars, which will no doubt keep growing, and she is the highest-paid entertainer on the planet. For those that haven't worked it out yet, I'm talking about Oprah. She owns her shit, in fact her shit is fuel for her growth. Hats off to that woman. Like her or not you can't deny she has done some amazing things with her adversity. I'm not a huge fan of her work but damn do I respect what she has done. She owns her shit and that is inspirational.

So, what are you going to do, anchor yourself down with blame or let that blame go and move forward?

Chapter 3: R

Moving onto R. I have chosen Reclaim, and the first thing we're going to reclaim is our movement.

Reclaiming your movement

We need movement, our physical and emotional wellbeing depends on it. As human beings, we have the most amazing gifts come as standard in our lives. The human brain is the most complex organ in the known universe with an almost limitless capacity to change and grow. To shape our very own reality how we see fit. It is that large and complex brain that enables us to move in such a variety of ways. We have more capacity for complex movement than any other organism, it truly is staggering seeing what people can do with effort and consistency. What do we do with that ability? We create all sorts of amazing technologies that make our life easier, just so we can sit on our arse on the sofa watching some life-wasting shit on TV, while eating stuff that isn't really food. It's no wonder that so many people are unhappy, unhealthy, and living in pain.

Pain is a sign that something needs to change. Unfortunately, it is seen by most in the modern world as an affliction instead of a sign. They live with it and hope it goes away, medicate it, or look to a doctor to save them. The thing that scares me is it's considered normal for people to go downhill, having pain and increasingly limited movement as they get older. Well it's not fucking normal. You should be able to move well right into old age. You will need to make an effort and use that movement though, it doesn't just happen. Use it or lose it, again. If you do lose it, well thankfully that doesn't mean you can't reclaim it. I know some people in their thirties blaming age for losing movement or being in pain and they give up, it's crazy. As soon as you start saying you are old, you are telling your brain you are old and it will listen. Never blame age or say you're feeling old. When you accept limitations, they become truth, fuck that shit. I went on a bit of a rant there, my bad.

The human brain is very energy-costly: it uses up around twenty percent of the body's overall energy expenditure. From a survival standpoint, being energy-costly isn't a good thing so our brains and bodies are always looking to save energy somewhere. A favourite tactic is to create habits and patterns that become automatic. The more automatic a task becomes, the less the brain needs to get involved in doing that task, it takes off some computational load. Whether it be a movement pattern, a psychological pattern or an emotional response, the principle is the same. It adapts, learns and looks to save energy.

We all know how habits can become problematic psychologically, and the same is true physically. I shall put this in the context of movement. Undoing dodgy movement patterns and getting people out of pain is a large part of what I do after all. Let's take sitting as an example, as it's something we all do, usually more than is healthy. During sitting, some muscles relax, some shorten, some lengthen, while others are more active in keeping us stable. The more we do it, the better we become at sitting. All those muscles become efficient at doing their jobs for that task and the pattern gets wired in. On the flip side, the better muscles get at doing those tasks, the worse they get at doing opposite tasks. The brain starts to forget those opposite movements. Some muscles get tighter, movement ability becomes lost and life starts to become smaller. Essentially, we start to lose territory in our own bodies. Pain is all too often coming along for the ride. This not only affects us physically but also emotionally.

Our psychological wellbeing is intimately tied to our body, the mind is the body and vice versa. Our posture and our mood go hand in hand, and if our body becomes restricted, so will our emotions. We all know when somebody is feeling low as their posture screams it. I want you to try a little experiment. All I want you to do is adopt the classic teenager posture, shoulders and chest slumped forward while looking down at the floor. Now pay attention to how you feel, try to feel happy, confident and strong. It doesn't happen, does it? Now try the opposite, sit or stand upright with your chest out, while your head and eyes are up. How do you feel? Do you feel lighter, stronger, more positive? This is a very simple demonstration of how our psychology and our physiology are linked. It is also a good little trick to get you in a better state that I shall expand on later, I promise.

How to change

I know, you want to know what can be done about the whole movement thing, or you should do anyway. There are a few simple pointers I can give. Now obviously everyone is different and some people need a bit more investigation, but I can't do anything about that without seeing people and this is a book, not a consultation after all! I'm just going to have to be general here. Almost everyone can increase their movement capacity in some way with a bit of effort and attention. The key is making a conscious effort to include some novel, complex movement training into your life. By complex I mean something that changes direction, levels, angles and has an element of learning to it. Earlier on I mentioned dance and martial arts, these are excellent examples, as is any gymnastic-type movement.

There is a whole movement of movement growing all over the world with people like Ido Portal leading the charge. I'm not suggesting you start busting out cartwheels in the gym or anything like that, but you can take small elements of those complex movements and tailor them to your needs. You don't have to completely change whatever exercise you do normally, just include a bit of complex, novel stuff in there somewhere. If you don't exercise then you'd better start. Exercise is not an option. Doing something more linear is good enough if you are unused to movement, build on it from there. We are essentially teaching our brain to move differently.

Let's not forget about stretching either. It is a wonderful addition to helping you move better when it's done right. The issue with a lot of stretching is it doesn't consider how the brain adapts, learns and looks to save energy. The key is to use stretching to increase muscle length for whatever is tight, then use that new length in some complex manner to teach the brain that it is usable. The brain will just go back to what it knows unless you teach it otherwise. I want to share with all you kiddywinks a simple tip on stretching for flexibility and movement that I use all the time. There's all sorts of neurological stuff going on that makes this method more effective than basic, static stretching. It's something known as "contract relax stretching." I'm going to assume that you have some knowledge of stretching, some that you have at least tried. You wouldn't be reading this if you didn't have at least a passing interest in moving better. If I'm wrong, then there is always YouTube. That's given me an idea, I will do some instructional type stuff on my YouTube for you guys and girls, so look out for that in the future.

So, start with stretches you know. Once you are in the position for whatever stretch you are doing, find the end range: that point where you can feel that the stretch won't go any further without forcing it. Make sure you maintain that position until you're finished with this stretching technique. Start to contract the muscle you are targeting, but not super hard—try fifty percent effort. Do that for five seconds, then relax the contraction but maintain the position, breathe out and try to increase the stretch if you can. If you can't increase the stretch, then just hold the position. Do whatever your muscles will let you do. Over time your body will get better at stretching. Repeat that process four times in total, four contractions of five seconds per stretch. That's it! Move on to the next stretch then go play with some new movement stuff. A quick word of warning though, after doing this kind of stretching don't go hammering the muscles away with heavy weights or push it hard. Coaxing is more effective and safer than forcing, you are teaching the brain something new after all.

My next bit of reclamation action is to reclaim your inner child.

Reclaim your inner child

There is a lot of crossover to the awareness section here—in fact this whole thing pretty much intertwines. As adults, we tend to take life all too seriously and put far too much importance into how other people may view us. Making us uptight and unhappy. Not only does being unhappy tend to lead to unhealthy life choices in a bid to distract us from that unhappiness, but it also has some direct effects on our physiology. Digestion and immune function can become compromised when people are chronically stressed and unhappy. Our health can take a hit. Remember the mind is the body, everything is linked here. Nothing happens in isolation.

Have you ever noticed how the most negative people in your life are plagued with movement issues, tight rigid bodies, faces that are older than their age, pain and illness? Look around, take note and you will see patterns. You will see the opposite is generally the case for truly happy people. I'm not talking about the fake happy people that relentlessly post positive quotes everywhere but when you see them their bodies tell a different story. The body never lies—it will tell you everything you need to know, you just need to be aware. Now I'm not saying we can never be sad or pissed off for whatever reason, life happens. I'm talking about the pervasive, chronic kind of stress and unhappiness that chips away at us long after the event, often for years or even a lifetime. The kind that ruins our quality of life and ultimately our health. I'm essentially talking about what happens when you attach yourself to thought. Remember that shit-stirring dickhead I spoke about earlier.

So, what does reclaiming your inner child have to do with all this? Well, to put it bluntly, everything. We have much to learn from the way children do things. Don't worry, I'm not suggesting you run around shitting your pants and dribbling, not in public anyway. What you choose to do in your own home is your business. I don't judge.

When kids are young they have a natural sense of wonder, they see adventure everywhere. There are no social boundaries, no worrying about how they look or sound to other people. They are open, naturally loving and fearless. We are only born with one innate fear and that is the fear of falling. We also have a reflexive reaction to sudden loud noises which some people consider a fear. Every other fear is learned from life experiences and people's upbringing. Fearful parents create fearful kids by constantly telling them to be careful and warning them of the perceived dangers in life.

Kids don't spend lots of time thinking about the past or worrying about the future. They are just living in the moment, for the most part. They'll be thinking a lot about the future when Christmas and birthdays are approaching, don't get me wrong, but otherwise they stay in the present. One of the greatest lessons we can learn from young children is how they approach learning. Kids love learning, they are fascinated by the world around them and want to know more. Let's take learning to walk for example. They're not put off by falling over, they keep trying and eventually they learn to walk.

Us adults on the other hand are pretty easily put off by falling, by perceived failures, particularly if there is an element to what other people might think about those failures. We either give up too easily or don't try at all, which ultimately is the biggest failure. If we thought like that as kids we would still be rolling around and shitting ourselves. Fear of failure is ultimately a fear of other people's opinions and I believe it is the single biggest reason the majority of the world is unhappy and doing work that they don't really love. Working for someone else's dream instead of their own.

How fear restricts us

How many people do you know that are unhappy with their work? Over ninety eight percent of the people I know, probably more. That is a scary thought, considering we spend most of our waking lives at work, traveling to and from work or thinking about work. If you don't love it then that adds up to a life lost to shit you hate. I think the internet is changing that number though. The world is at our finger tips and we have much more control and access to information than ever before. Pre-internet days, information was just there for those who could afford it or did well in the school system. Neither of those things were me, that's for sure. So, thanks internet. Big love.

We live in a time of vast opportunity and have the power to shape our destinies like never before, if we can just drop this bullshit idea that other people's opinions matter. It is crippling. Fear of failing, of other people's opinions, is also what keeps so many people out of shape and unhealthy. I've lost count of the amount of times I've heard someone say they can't join a gym, go to an exercise class, take up some kind of sport, martial art, or activity until they've lost some weight first or are fitter. Which wouldn't be so bad if they actually then got fitter and did the thing, but I'm yet to see that happen.

They are literally letting what other may people think stop them from ever starting. So, they stay at home, slipping further into weight gain and poor health and unhappiness. For me, if I see someone who is out of shape walk into the gym or into a class I get excited. In my head, I think "Yes, go on son (or girl), you took that first big scary step, big fucking respect." Everyone is there for the same reason, ultimately: they want to feel good. In the highly unlikely event that a tiny minority may judge you for taking that first step, that says more about them than you anyway. I mean how insecure and unhappy would you have to be to not support someone trying to improve their health and happiness? That's certainly not somebody whose opinion is worth taking notice of—fuck what they think. Even if there is someone out there like that, they probably wouldn't actually say it to your face, so you wouldn't even know.

Sometimes that insecure and unhappy person may be someone you know, possibly a family member. We all have those negative people around us somewhere that only see the shit in a situation. They will be negative no matter what but that is their problem, you don't have to make it yours. Now if I was to say to you "I want you to throw away your health, your happiness, your dreams, basically your life, so that some unhappy and insecure people can't judge you," would that sound like a good trade off, a life for somebody else's insecurities? Fucking sign me up, I'll take two, what a bargain. This isn't just about health and fitness, it's about life. Your life is yours, not anybody else's, so live it by your standards, your morals, your heart's guidance, your truth.

We've established that young kids don't care what the world thinks around them, they just get on and play. Something we could all learn from. What else can we learn from them? Have you ever noticed how kids don't doubt their abilities? They're always saying things like "Watch me run really fast", "I can jump really high", "I drew this". They don't doubt what they can do, in fact they are showing it with excitement and pride. Not like most of us adults who tend to be riddled with self-doubt. Which again, is just another expression of fear of other people's opinions.

Something else we can learn from kids that can add so much to our lives is taking time out to play, to be silly, to have fun. Unsurprisingly this is tied in with other people's opinions, again. We stop ourselves from really letting loose because of what other people may think. We may only be able to let loose a bit with the help of alcohol or drugs, which come with their own cost, sometimes a very heavy cost. Any fun experienced like that is superficial and unfulfilling at best. At worst it is destructive, be it to yourself, your relationships, those around you at the time or all of the above. Personally, I have nothing against drugs and alcohol or any other way people chose to spend their leisure time. The issue lays in the relationship with that substance or pastime, not the thing itself. If you are relying on it to have fun, let loose and escape, then there is a problem. Whatever that thing may be, it could be anything.

Having a sense of fun in your life is so important that without it our health and happiness is going to pay the price. Nobody wants to be unhappy and unhealthy, it's hardly a lifelong ambition. So, go out and find something that is fun, silly and childish, in a good way. Play on some swings, go to one of those trampoline parks that have been popping up recently, climb a tree, dance, play with a yoyo. You are only limited by your imagination. I recently attempted to climb a tree for the first time in over 20 years. The keyword being 'attempted'. As a man that weighs around 106kg, I found it, shock horror, considerably more difficult than when I was younger and much lighter. It is now part of my week to dedicate some time to trying to climb trees. I may look mental to onlookers but I don't give a shit. It's fun, it's really challenging physically, it totally counts as complex novel movement and it forces me to be very present, in the moment. That is some excellent boxes ticked. Shall we move on?

Chapter 4: E

E is for express: express your creativity and express your truth. Going in order then...

Creativity

Why is it even important? Well, creativity is what sets us apart from all other life on this planet, we are creators. We have seemingly endless possibilities for our creativity. Words, music, art, dance, fashion, food, martial arts, technology, the list goes on. Humanity is built on constant, ever-evolving creativity. It is my belief that having some sort of creativity is crucial for human happiness. I don't know anyone who is truly happy without it, do you?

When we are denied that creativity we become unhappy, depressed, frustrated and life gets messy. It was a big problem for me and many other kids in school. As I grew up on a council estate, as working class as you can get, where the choice of schools wasn't a choice. I went to a normal secondary school where pupils are prepared for real life, or in other words trained to become an obedient consumerist workforce. That's the role of your average school. The education provided in higher, elite schools is very different. There they are prepared for life in higher roles, so they don't need to learn the same stuff as those lower down the food chain. They too will still be expected to fit into a certain way of thinking, so I would no doubt have done badly at school no matter where I went, or my economic background.

Now I can't really blame the teachers as that's all they know—they are bound and educated by that very same system. Unfortunately for my teachers and my mum, I could not be tamed. For years I thought I was just a naughty little shit who went off the rails (and go off the rails I did). Thankfully I know now that my "bad behaviour" was a symptom, a reaction to being boxed in by our education system. I have always been the same with work as well, which is why I now work for myself, doing my own thing, following my heart, doing what I think is right and not what is imposed on me.

My work allows me a ton of creative discovery. It is the only way I can function. Without it I'd be hiding in drugs, alcohol, junk food, or all three. I'm not saying that working for yourself is for everyone though. I know it isn't. What I'm talking about having a creative outlet. Whatever it is that inspires you, that you enjoy. It could be anything. For me, I love Brazilian jujitsu—it is exercise, complex movement and allows so much creativity. It ticks all the boxes for me. Add to that the fact that my work is creative too, and it's no wonder I'm a pretty happy guy. I'm not suggesting my life is a bed of roses but the good far outweighs the bad and that's a lot more than most people can say. I have tipped the scales in my favour.

Anyway, this isn't about me, this is about you. If you don't already have a way to express your creativity, then you'd better find a way. Maybe it's something that you used to do before being a grown-up got in the way, or maybe it's something you've always wanted to try. The chances are you already know what it is. Just give yourself permission to do it. Creativity is a human need.

Live your truth

Expressing your truth and being true to who you are can be scary. Again, it is something that is often discouraged in school, and sometimes by parents who have forgotten what it is like to live their own truth. My personal favourite and an all-too-common occurrence is when parents or guardians push their version of the truth onto their kids, and that version of truth isn't even the parents in the first place!

It absolutely happens in most workplaces as well, particularly in the corporate world. Fairly recently, to the time of writing this anyway, I was in talks with one of the top hotels in central London who wanted to hire me to come in and do some work in their spa. Part of what I do, what I'm known for, is my work as an advanced movement neurology (AMN) practitioner. It is a therapeutic system created from the genius mind of David Fleming. If you're reading this Dave, I fucking love you. It is based on how the brain and the body communicate and has very far reaching applications. It can do so much: getting people out of pain and moving better, improving mental performance, coordination, recovery from strokes, brain injuries, sleep problems, digestive issues, and even deeper health issues. There is a lot that can be done as ultimately the brain tells the body what to do. I have yet to find the boundaries of what can be done, I'm always looking!

One of my favourite clients was an eight-year old boy. He suffered with dyspraxia to the point that he could not do anything that involved any kind of coordination. I remember when his mum first brought him in to me. His whole posture was slumped forward, he was constantly fidgeting and could not make eye contact. One of the tests I used involved him being on all fours and doing specific movements. When I asked him to get into the position, he fell over before we got to the actual test bit. Not even being able to get on all fours was much more than just a little coordination problem. This obviously affected his confidence and overall quality of life as he couldn't play with the other kids like they did, which was something I could really relate to. Nowadays he is running, climbing things, playing football, going to trampoline parks and doing all the things an active kid should do. His mum sent me pictures of him racing in sports day, all proud and I fully admit, it did make me shed a single manly tear when I saw those pics. The change in him was dramatic, he is now a confident and active boy—much better than I ever was.

Back to this hotel then. They wanted to be the first hotel to have an AMN practitioner onboard in the world. After a couple of meetings at this hotel and a demonstration of how I work, they started trying to box me in. Wanting me to fit the treatment into a shorter time frame, make it more structured and less intuitive while deliberately only addressing a couple of things during the sessions and leaving the person wanting more. I can see that from a business point of view this means more through the door, it does however make it more like a conveyer belt which I am not down with. The system itself is very intuitive and relies completely on how the client is responding to the techniques as feedback. It is that very intuitive nature that appeals so much to me. Now the money was good, the hourly rate was double what I was charging at the time but I was having a dilemma. Deep down I knew I couldn't work like that, I knew I would be unhappy. Also, I'm in this game to help, not to partially help some people so this hotel can get more people through the door.

At the time of writing this there are fewer than twenty people worldwide at the top end of the AMN tree, and it was nearer half that at the time. I was one of the very first and I couldn't justify going through all that learning, knowledge and the experience I had gained just to cut the system down for short-term financial gain. Not only that, they would've expected me to behave in a certain way. Definitely no swearing and dancing around like a twat, which are both things I tend to do a lot of. Well that was me out. I sent them an email declining and chose to put all my energy into my business, where I can carry on being me, living my truth. There really was no choice. I can only be me and have lost a lot of jobs because people wanted me to do things different. Once I came to the realisation that living by my code, my values, my heart was the only way, life became so much more fun. No more pretending, no more being a square peg in a round hole, trying to round off my shoulders to fit in.

You are unique, there is nobody on this planet like you, even if you're a twin. You are you. Your hopes, dreams, passions, experiences are yours. Embrace it, own your shit, be you. If you think of the biggest names in Hollywood, the superstars, they aren't always the most talented, the most diverse in skillset. What they all have in common is they are themselves within a role, it is not their ability to act a certain way, it is the ability to make that character theirs, they own it.

Now I want to put a bit of a disclaimer here. There are people out there, and I'm sure you will have met them, that say they are just being honest, being real and speaking truth but actually, are just using it as an excuse to be rude and nasty to people. There is difference between living your truth and just behaving like a wanker. That kind of behaviour is just a defence mechanism to keep people from getting too close, deter people from messing with them, or to hide their vulnerability. There is an old Chinese saying that I love and it is relevant to that type of person. It is "the loudest dog in the room is the weakest dog in the room." Living your truth isn't about walking round telling that truth to everyone you meet. That would be totally impractical and cause way too much conflict.

We have all been hurt in life. In reaction to the painful events in our lives, we tend to adopt behaviours and mechanisms to prevent similar occurrences from happening again. Our brain wants to protect us from harm, physical and emotional. As a result, it will make subconscious adaptations. It is very much part of our evolution. As the modern world has moved on at a pace that far outmatches evolutionary development, we run into problems. Our evolutionary traits don't fit this environment too well. We have a primal brain and body that's trying to get by in this fast-paced modern world and failing for the most part. There are countless unhappy people being unhealthy and feeling a bit lost. This is why this book exists. I developed a whole host of behaviours throughout my life that didn't do me a lot of good at the time. Saying that though, they bought me here and I learned a lot in the process so I guess they ultimately were useful, once acknowledged. Those many behaviours were too numerous to go into here. All I will say is I was very skilled at being a messed-up fuckwit, a master of the ancient art of fuckwittery.

When living your truth, you will need to be honest with yourself and do bit of soul searching. Is it your truth, is it a mechanism, or are you playing up to somebody else's expectations? It is about living life to your values, your heart and not being moulded to suit other people's agendas. To quote The Bible, which is something I rarely do as I'm not religious in that sense, "The truth shall set you free." Jesus said that, apparently. It probably sounded very different in Hebrew though.

Owning your body

While we're on the subject of living your truth, I want to talk about the physical side of that: owning your physical state, embodying your essence, making your body yours, and being confident in your own skin. When somebody truly owns their shit, they stand out, they shine. You notice them when they enter a room. They may not be the best looking or wear the best clothes but they are extremely attractive because they own it, they have impact. Just so we're clear, I'm not necessarily talking about sexual attraction. I mean your eyes are drawn to them, they attract your attention over everyone else in the room. When you are true to yourself, living your truth, it gives you this kind of quality. There is a certain amount of confidence that comes with living your truth. Confidence, as the saying goes, is king.

There are strategies that you can use to put yourself into this confident state at will. As physiology and psychology are intimately linked, you can use your physiology to put you in a better, higher state. The simplest way is to change your posture, how you are sitting or standing. If you raise your posture tall—chest up, shoulders back and look upwards—you will feel very different than if you're slouched forward looking down. This is the very same technique I talked about back in the reclaim your movement section. If you add a smile in there, it helps you along your way.

The great thing about this technique is it's subtle, you can do it anywhere unnoticed. You can add a phrase to it, some self-talk to help you feel empowered. It can be in your head or out loud, depending on where you are or how much you care what those around you are thinking (I hope not too much by now). My personal phrase when I need to flick that switch is "Come on motherfucker." I am a massive potty mouth though, so you may want to choose something more appropriate to you. If you really want to ramp it up, then get dynamic. Bounce on the spot, punch the air, open your arms wide, chuck in some star jumps, basically move with a bit of energy.

Using your physical body to change emotional state has been used by many of the world's top performers in various fields. It is widely used in sports, music, acting and public speaking. We can use it too to perform at our best. It can be a high-pressure environment like an interview or important meeting. Maybe it's a difficult conversation you know you need to have with someone or you need to raise your state to get out of an emotional slump and move forward. Experiment to see what sort of movement works for you. Once you have something that you're happy with, you can anchor it to a song you like that makes you feel motivated. All you need to do is play it while you use your chosen techniques to get into a good state. Repeat the process a few times.

Now when you hear that song in the future it should help put you in a better state without having to do all the physical stuff if you're in public.

Another very powerful anchor you can use is smell. The olfactory system (our sense of smell) is the only one of our senses that fires directly into the emotional centres of our brain, making it very powerful indeed. Can you recall a time when you've smelled something for the first time in years and it takes you right back to that place? Many businesses take advantage of this. Supermarkets and bakers pump that smell of fresh bread out in the air all the time to set people off. Restaurants try to make sure their food can be smelled outside. Casinos and posh hotels have certain smells pumped around them to help put people in a good state. You can use it too as an anchor. Just do everything you did before to change your state and include a specific fragrance in there. Make sure the fragrance isn't super common, you don't want to be running into that smell all the time. You want to keep it just for you, to help trigger that higher state. It could be an essential oil or a perfume or aftershave. I use a small scented candle that lives in my work bag and comes out whenever that switch needs to be flicked. Yes, I probably do look a bit strange randomly sniffing a candle in public places. The more astute of you will have worked by now out that I don't give a shit.

Chapter 5: T

Moving on to T then...

Take control of your information.

This is a simple concept that can be applied to every aspect of your life. Our neurology functions on an information and communication basis. The brain is receiving information constantly. This happens externally from the environment and internally from us. Based on that information, our brain tells the body to what do. So, what do I mean by information? Well, everything. I'll break it up into a few categories for you. This list is by no means complete though.

Nutrition

Nutrition is information. The food and drink we take in. It all has something to say to our brain and body. Shit food is shit information and you will get a shit response. That being said, there are foods that you may think are good for you that your body doesn't like. Everyone is different, there is no cookie cutter diet for everyone. There are some things that are universally considered crap, but the rest is down to how your body handles it. We've all been there when we've eaten something and shortly after started feeling crap. It may be brain fog, lethargy, headaches, breathing issues, bloating and sometimes a closer relationship with the toilet. It can also affect your sleep patterns. Sometimes it can be less of a physical feeling—the wrong food choices can affect your mood as well. If you've ever switched from feeling OK to suddenly feeling irritable, snappy, and finding yourself a lot less tolerant, the answer could very well lay in what you've eaten. Next time it happens, backtrack and see if you can work out what set you off.

If you really want to be clever about it you can keep a food and mood diary, track it all and make correlations. It's a great tool that can have a profound impact on your life. Personally, it was life changing for me when I did this. As I'm nice I shall tell you quickly how to do it and I'll include a PDF for you right here.

https://docs.wixstatic.com/ugd/c10bc6_07cddf932047410e991480a7d6217eb7.pdf

In the PDF you will see that I have included sections for four meals. Feel free to apply that to however many meals you eat a day.

- For each meal, you will have three sections. The first section is food, unsurprisingly. The key to this section is details. For example, if you had a chicken sandwich, you would put down the kind of bread, the spread, if it's chicken breast or thigh. You get the idea, the more details the better. All fluids and supplements should be noted down too.

- The other sections are to be filled out around forty-five mins to an hour after eating. One is for energy levels and focus. Do you feel sharp, tired, foggy, clear or whatever?

- The other section would be for your mood. You would put here how you feel: happy, depressed, angry, calm, irritable, sad, or whatever you're feeling.

- Over time you will learn exactly what your brain and body like, function well on and what's not so good for them. Be aware, it is important that you are patient and consistent with this. It takes a while to get the hang of, but it is totally worth the effort. When your body consistently gets what it wants, it goes a long way to performing at a higher level. You will have a better understanding of you and that is invaluable.

Exercise and movement

The kind of exercise you engage in, or not as the case may be, is giving your brain and body information to which there will be a response. If you're doing very little, then your body will adapt the muscles to the positions you are in the most. I used sitting down as an example earlier—movement becomes restricted and pain is often not far away. The same is true if you are doing the same thing repeatedly without any real variation. The muscles that get used the most start to tighten while those that get neglected tend to be longer and weaker, creating imbalances that, again, may well contribute to pain at some point. Just think of someone that loves working their chest more than anything else, their body shape is obvious. Tight chest and rounded shoulders, with elbows pointing out to the sides rather than pointing backwards. The knuckle dragger look. We are literally shaped by what we do (and think) the most.

The most important thing with exercise is first to do something you enjoy so that it is sustainable. There is no point doing stuff you hate. Then I would look at variety within that or something that complements it. Remember the brain loves complex movement, include some somewhere. Obviously, all of you sporty types will already have your sports that you do, so for you guys it's about doing stuff that allows you longevity in your chosen activity. This is where a well-structured weights training program comes into its own. It enables your body to cope with the demands of the activity and should, if designed correctly, deal with any imbalances that come from doing the same activity repeatedly. So, no cookie cutter programs here, it's worth getting a professional to do that for you. Someone that will take some sort of training history into account. Having your sporting years cut short from badly planned or lack of strength training is all too common. If you love what you do then take steps to ensure you can do it for as long as possible. Bit of a no brainer really.

Relationships

This one is a sensitive subject but very important. Ignore it at your peril. This isn't just about significant others. Family, friends, and colleagues all count too. If the people you are around the most are largely having negative conversations—bitching, moaning, blaming, being judgemental and generally putting a downer on things—it's a problem. It will be unconsciously shaping the way you think and feel. Whether you are aware of it or not, your subconscious mind sees and hears everything. Misery loves company, as the saying goes. Well so does positivity, thankfully!

Have you ever noticed how miserable people flock together? Well so do positive people that are interested in growth. Now I understand that we can't just cut some relationships out of our lives and that telling people to piss off all the time will do more harm than good. What we can do though is change how we relate with those people that we can't walk away from. Change the things we talk about in order to guide them in a new direction as best we can.

We can also build new relationships with more positive people by actively seeking them out. If you can't find any in your vicinity then there is always the internet, there are plenty of groups and forums of likeminded people or inspirational people you can follow. As we grow, those old negative relationships should naturally break away or change with you, to some degree. There is an important side note on all this, something that I believe many people go wrong with when giving this advice. Please take into account that there will be times your loved ones will need you to listen, love, and support them through hardship. Walking away from that would be no good for them or you. Being there for people is part of what makes us human. Honour that while still building your positive network around them. The aim is to get more positive interactions than negative, and therefore tip the scales in your favour.

Media

Now this one is massive, it's pervasive and it sneaks under the radar. I'm including media in all its forms from newspapers, magazines, books, TV, radio and, thanks to technological advances, social media that we carry around with us all day, every day. I'll start with newspapers or news sources in general. Many people start and end the day by checking out current affairs from whatever their preferred source is. I'm sure the observant of you will have noticed that it is always heavily skewed towards the negative, all doom and gloom. For some reason fear sells much more than hope and positivity, fuck knows why. It's not going to set you up for a good day and you certainly don't want that being the last thing your brain sees before you go to bed.

TV. Now here is a nasty fucker. The majority of TV is negative and full of conflict. Soaps, dramas, reality TV, and don't get me started on that toxic bastard Jeremy Kyle. It puts me in a negative state just thinking about it. People spend hours at a time in front of the TV absorbing all this stuff and having it shape our thoughts. Fortunately, since the internet we also have much more access to different things, so we can actively seek out more positive, interesting things, if we care to look. The world is at our finger tips. We have podcasts, video streaming, audio books, or you could even go old school and pick up one of those paper books.

Social media is sneaky and addictive. The amount of time spent checking phones is huge. It is largely unconscious as well, grabbing the phone without thinking about it, and then our minds are at the mercy of what is on Facebook or whatever we are using. How many times have you scrolled down and ended up in a bad mood after reading the endless stream of crap people post or share? Fortunately, we now have the option to hide people without deleting them, at least with Facebook, so that saves a lot of potential grief, particularly if it is a family member. I suggest you make use of that feature. As for other platforms, well you will just have to make sure you follow more positive than negative pages and people. Keep on tipping those scales.

Personally, I like to start the day on something positive. I like motivational things early, it sets the day up right for me and gathers momentum when done consistently. I also like to end the day on a positive note, reading or listening to something that will leave me in a good frame of mind before I sleep. The very first and the last thing I do each day is write down my goals in life, I have a book purely for that one thing. Another great tool is a gratitude book, where you write down a set number of things that you are grateful for each night before bed. That way you go to sleep in a good frame of mind. Your mind is going to get programmed whether you like it or not. You can take control and do it yourself or let the world around you do it for you. No contest, really is it?

The quality of your life is dependent on the quality of your information. Take control of your information and guide your life in the direction you want.

Chapter 6: H

The last letter is H. It stands for Help. Help others.
Essentially, try to do some good in the world. As a
species, we are not solitary animals, we are pack
animals. We live in herds, or as people like to call
them, communities. Communities rely on each
other, that is the nature of community, and that is
the nature of us. There are very few people that live
a truly isolated existence. Unless you are one of
those rare hermits, your life will be dependent on
many things from other people.

Consider the clothes you wear, your home, your
car, the roads you drive on, this book, the food you
eat, your gas and electricity, the internet. Basically,
everything you own and use has been made and
supplied by other people. You can dig down as far
as you want on this.

Let's take my laptop that I'm sat here writing this
up on, for example. For me to be able have this at
my fingertips, there will have been so many people
involved in the design, manufacture, packaging,
transport and sale before it gets to me. Not only

that, people will have been involved in the building of the road network, the manufacture of that transport, building my home and everything in it that I use so I can type this. All those people will have been fed to exist, they will have been taught how to do their jobs by other people. Their parents will have had sex, their grandparents will have had sex, my parents had sex, your parents had sex, yes yours, more than once and probably in different positions. They enjoyed it too, at least one of them did.

Human life is interconnected, in fact all life is interconnected, we are not separate from the flow of life, we are life. When you help others in life, you're helping life itself which means you are helping you, because you are life. OK, let's not get tied up in this too much, I'm getting a bit carried away there, I'll tone down my inner hippy!

Why help people?

Helping other people is important for two reasons:

One, the knock-on effect it has on other people can be massive. If you do something good for someone, putting them in a good place, then how they then interact with other people will be from a place of positivity, which can have a chain reaction of good shit that spreads out far and wide. The opposite is also true, if you upset someone that can shade how they interact with people and so on. We've all been in a bad mood from something, maybe somebody at work, some rude service in a shop, abusive drivers etc. We've gone home and maybe snapped at our partners, family members, kids, the dog. You get the idea. Now I'm not suggesting you become passive and take shit from people, nobody should be a doormat, I'm just suggesting you be more mindful of your interactions. You could help someone out one day who goes on to do wonderful things and comes back to thank you with some grand gesture, you never know.

So, we have the knock-on effect as one reason, what's the second reason?

Well do it because it makes you feel good. The smile on a child's face, someone's gratitude, seeing somebody achieve something that you've helped in, they all make us feel good directly. Sometimes you won't get anything back other than a sense of knowing you did something good.

I'm going to admit something here that my ego tried resisting for quite some time. My self-value is completely tied to helping others. If I felt that I wasn't doing any good in the world, I would become depressed. Inevitably I would try to self-medicate with drugs and alcohol to dull my emptiness, my sense of no purpose. "What's the point?" was a phrase I would use a lot. Some people hide themselves in material objects and distractions to hide that sense. For me it was always drugs. Looking back on my life, I now realise that the only jobs I could ever hold down, for any length of time had helping people at their core. It gave me a sense of purpose and enjoyment. Stick me in a warehouse, office job, or building site and I wouldn't make it past two weeks. It felt too much like work. Saying that though, those roles are helping people too, I just didn't see it at the time. Personally, I need to feel that direct sense of helping and connection which is why I do what I do. Working in a hospital I had that sense, and working in a school too. The many years I spent as a doorman in clubs and bars gave me that sense, even though most of the people didn't see it at the time. There have been many occasions where I've saved people's skin and they don't even know it. Now days I'm very happy to say there are no more late nights, there's no more violence and no more trying to argue logically with drunk people, which is scientifically impossible. My work is now based around things like writing this. Helping guide people through their mind and body so they can take ownership of the vehicle they live in, getting people out of pain and moving better. Nobody wants to feel trapped in their body, or their mind for that matter. Not that those things happen separately, as I'm sure you are aware by now.

Helping is a service

From a business point of view, the more people you serve and help, the more you earn. The correlation is direct. The biggest businesses have the biggest reach "serving" the most people. You may not personally agree with that business's methods or want their version of help but a lot of people do, or they wouldn't exist. An example that I was given that changed the way I looked at service is Premier League footballers. At the top end, one of the highest paid footballers (or soccer players) right now, while I'm writing this anyway, is Paul Pogba. He makes two hundred and ninety thousand pounds a week. You heard me right, that's £290,000. A week. That will be directly proportionate to how well he serves his club, his performances, the merchandising and millions of fans worldwide that he entertains. Entertainment and inspiration is the service for the fans. Just as it is for any athlete, musician, movie star and nowadays, social media stars. It may seem like they get paid a disproportionate amount but the amount of people they are touching is huge. You can follow that logic easily to any successful business or individual. So financially, the more people you can help, the better off you will be. This isn't a business section by the way, I'm just making a point about helping others.

Purpose (and crabs)

Helping others is what takes a purpose from you to something bigger than you. When your sense of purpose comes from something that is bigger than you, the fulfilment you feel will be greater. Not only that, but the lengths you are willing go for that purpose will also be greater. You would no doubt go to the ends of the earth to save a loved one who was in pain, much further than if it was just you. If your business or career goals are about something bigger than you, you will fight through a lot more of the shit than you would if it was just about you. It makes your drive and motivation much greater which in turn will allow your achievements to be greater. There is no limit to where purpose outside of yourself can take you. Happiness cannot exist without a sense of purpose.

There are plenty of people out there, who have outwardly successful lives, who inside are suffering from a lack of purpose and meaning. Living a selfish life will ultimately lead to unhappiness so it is self-defeating anyway, like the crabs in a bucket scenario. For those of you that have never heard of crabs in a bucket, I will tell you all about it. If you put a single crab in a bucket, that crab will (assuming it is a decent size) usually be able to work out how to get out. If you put more crabs in, something very interesting happens. When a crab tries to make a break for it, the others will drag it back. It goes on like that, crabs clambering over each other to get out while pulling each other down. Driven by complete self-preservation, they all eventually die, ironically. We are not crabs, we can choose different. Helping others is helping yourself, the best way to be selfish. The world around you and the world inside you will become a better place for helping others.

Congratulations!

That's it folks, you've made it to the end. Well done. Thanks for reading, I am truly grateful. You are helping me in my mission to help undo the shit the modern world does to us. The whole point of this book is to help you function a little better in your life. You could be in business, high-performance sports, sales, teaching, a full-time parent or literally anything else that a human can do with their time. It really doesn't matter what you do—you will always do it better if you look after yourself and do it with love. We live in a 'more is better' world where we're encouraged to constantly grind. Busyness is considered a virtue and everyone wants more productivity. The irony is that being busy doesn't make you more productive, quite the opposite in fact. It is the space where the magic arises. That is where we heal, where we grow, where we find our flow. Whenever someone learns to manage their own health and happiness, the world becomes a tiny bit of a better place. The love starts to grow. So, do your bit, for yourself, for those around you and the world.

It's up to you now, it's always been up to you.

Big punkass love,

Gareth

P.S. If you've learned anything useful in here then you might want to check out my site or Facebook pages for future endeavours. There are many plots cooking in my head.

www.garethriddy.com

www.facebook.com/TheGarethRiddy/ My therapy based page

www.facebook.com/GarethRiddyTheMan/ My just me page, thoughts, book stuff and who knows what else.

Acknowledgements

There are so many people that have helped me on my journey through life. There is a strong possibility that I will miss some people out. If that's you, my bad, I love you. I'll start with the one, my wife Nicola. The only woman to not try and change me. Your love, endless support and belief in me are truly a blessing. Being with you has allowed me to grow. I am me because you are you. Fuck knows what sort of fraggle I would be without you. My gran for saving my skin and being a sanctuary, without you I doubt I would have made it into my twenties. My Aunt Sue, for being the biggest rock of the family. For all those times you took me on holiday because mum couldn't afford it and for putting up with my dickish behaviour. The world needs more people with your strength. Dad, I know you did your best. I am so happy to have you back in my life. Bink, you showed me that there was more to life, that I could be more. It just took me a while to get that. Mark Adams who taught me to look deeper and to think outside the box, you made me want to be a better trainer. Dave Fleming, well what can I say, my world was never the same again.

You are the single biggest influence in my education, what I learned from you changed everything and you laugh at my jokes. Luke Sherrell for being the business head to get Dave's stuff out of his head and to me. Also for all the help with marketing this. Andy Harrington, although I don't personally know you, the effect you had on me is massive. Attending your Power to Achieve event and doing the repatterning process opened me right up to my truth, I am a better human being because of you. Rachel for literally saving my life with CPR, I simply can't thank you enough to do it justice. Natasha Jones, your advice rocked. This book grew because of you. Linda for all your help with the website, book design and for always being there to take the piss like true friends do. Chris jones for some fine photography and the many hours we spent consuming chicken wings over the years. Coach Katherine for keeping my head in the game. Phil Else, the greatest martial arts coach I have ever had the honour to learn from. I miss us trying to choke the shit out of each other and me usually losing. Everyone I have stepped on a matt or in a cage with, so many lessons. Every doorman or woman that has been by my side over the years.

Even those few that ran away, I learned from you too. All my family and friends, you all have had your part to play. My most painful clients that gave me the biggest professional lessons and tested me.

Finally, this book, my work and my life is dedicated to my mum. Your love and your pain drives me. R.I.P.

I love you.

Finally, if you liked the stuff in this little book, please leave me a review on amazon. It helps my book's visibility on the site so hopefully I can help more people. Ultimately the whole point of this book is it's my own way of trying to do some good in the world and trying put a smile in more places. We need more smiles and love in the world

.

This book was written with love by Gareth Riddy

Edited and made to look like a grown-up book by Jake Waller

Designed and jazzed up by James Hood